Praise for Rain / Dweller

"I really enjoyed reading these poems and, because I felt driven forward by them, read them all in one sitting. Part of the loveliness of it for me was the expectation of arriving at yet another arresting line—of being brought to a halt by something piercingly true expressed finely. I was also captivated by Risa Denenberg's contemplation of that place where our most fundamental concerns as humans—love, death, aging, sadness, and the mystery of it all—meet the natural world. I felt myself in the presence of a great honesty about things that matter, and in particular responded to the idea that, despite our existential plight—maybe even because of it—life is a thing of great beauty."

  —David Guterson, author of *Snow Falling on Cedars*

"'It's too easy to look away, say nothing,' Risa Denenberg tells us in what could be the mantra of a book that steadfastly refuses to do either – a book that takes hold of the reader's gaze and directs our looking at loss and hardship both personal and global, human and animal, physical and emotional. From apocalyptic kitten sonnets to a piercing series of selfie poems, Denenberg's wry, straightforward, penetrating voice is rebuke, meditation, and celebration all at once, gnarly and braided as the beloved trees she offers prayers for. 'Finding something to live for / is my talent, this small raft,' Denenberg writes, and indeed amidst the sorrow, she keeps hold of us, pointing to the everyday, essential miracles of sustenance and small things, of clouds, of the simple and necessary plan to sing, as she does with fierceness and compassion, in gladness."

  —Corrie Williamson, author of
  The River Where You Lost My Name

"In this honest and unflinching collection, Denenberg gives us poems that look at hard topics like extinction, climate change, aging, and loss, and tempers them with tenderness, vulnerability, beauty, and delight—delight in the moon, the face of a pet, powdered snow on cedars. Inviting us to grow 'passably fond of rain,' *Rain Dweller* teaches us how 'Every day, the clouds amaze.'"

—Rena Priest, Washington State Poet Laureate, 2021-2023, and author of *Patriarchy Blues*

RAIN/DWELLER

RAIN/DWELLER

poems

Risa Denenberg

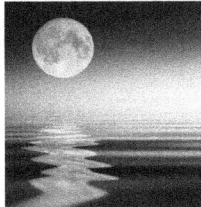

MoonPath Press

Poetry
ISBN 978-1-936657-73-5

Cover art: *Vernal Water* (2009) digital photograph by Jayne
Marek

Author photo by Ronda Piszk Broatch

Book design by Tonya Namura, using Minion Pro.

MoonPath Press, an imprint of Concrete Wolf Poetry Series,
is dedicated to publishing the finest poets
living in the U.S. Pacific Northwest.

MoonPath Press
PO Box 445
Tillamook, OR 97141

MoonPathPress@gmail.com

http://MoonPathPress.com

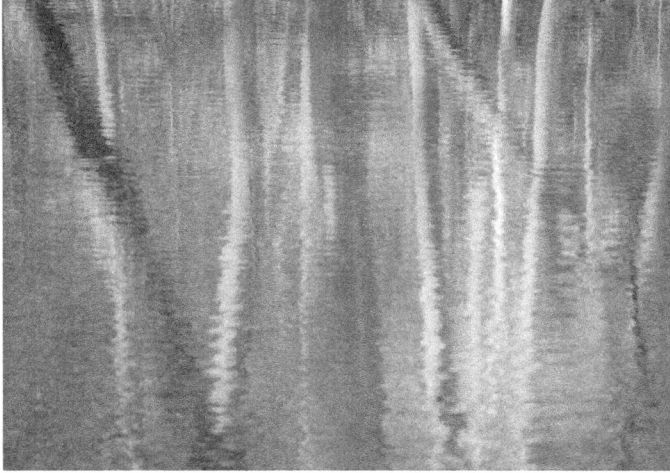

For Yann, Dilan, Skyler, & Lucas.
We did not do enough, sorry doesn't cut it,
and now it's up to you.
May you walk gently upon the earth.

Table of Contents

Little we see in Nature that is ours;
We have given our hearts away, a sordid boon!
This Sea that bares her bosom to the moon;
The winds that will be howling at all hours,
And are up-gathered now like sleeping flowers;
For this, for everything, we are out of tune;
It moves us not.

—William Wordsworth,
The World Is Too Much with Us

Nonetheless I honor your name
for allowing me tenancy on this, your firmament,
and I accept its provision as my lot.

—Campbell McGrath,
The Mercy Supermarket

Old Trees, Old Lovers: A Postscript

I dream of trees: far-flung sisters.
Their future resides beyond our ruin.

I love what is gnarly, what is braided—
banyans and mangroves, the hued peeling bark
    of madronas—
in the same way I love my worn, battered boots.
I know my position. I've unwound my watch.

Kismet flickers in the distance. I turn to you for succor,
but you've disappeared. We're a couple of old shrubs now,
    slowly dying.
But look, over there: flocks of fledglings.

Let us now cede this land to trees.
Let them lean towards one another,
stand their ground in squalls, sway in zephyrs.

I pray they endure without us.

RAIN/DWELLER

one

Extremophile

Born in the full darkness of permafrost placenta, I was
installed with others' memories. Packed to deliver the
genetic goods, then swept aside, buried deep within
memory itself. Sutured into a sleeping bag of frozen
tundra, I shun life in a temperate zone. I align only
with rare creatures: lemmings and voles, the occasional
snowbird that subsists on lichens. And though I vaguely
recall another time and place, I cannot say what I'm
doing here, sewing buttons on red shirts for dead
soldiers.

How Two Trees Become a Forest

after Arthur Sze

A teacher draws Chinese characters on the chalkboard
to show how two trees become a forest. Chalk is soft
white limestone composed of the shells of foraminifers.
A student looks up the Chinese character for shell. An
Afghani schoolgirl covers her head and walks to the
schoolhouse with broken windows. She tells her teacher
she hopes to become a doctor. I bring soup to a neighbor
who tells me she hopes to die soon. The girl on the radio
sings, *my body's in trouble*. I wonder will I die alone. A
lonely boy pauses in front of a girl sketching a forest of
firs and yews. Their branches barely move in the humid
haze of noon. An infant grabs the wooden slats of her
crib and pulls herself up to cry out for her mother. I
think how much is lost without these signs to guide us.
Foraminifers are single-celled amoebae. The foramen
ovale is a hole in the heart that must close at birth.

Ice Would Suffice

How swift, how far
the sea
carries a body from shore.

Empires fail, species are lost,
spotted frogs
and tufted puffins forsaken.

After eons of fauna and flora, hominids have stood
for mere years,
baffled brains atop battered shoulders.

In a murky blanket of heavens,
an icy planet
made of diamond spins.

Our sun winks like the star
it was
billions of years ago, without ambition.

We bury bodies in shallow dirt, heedless of lacking space
or how long
our makeshift planet will host us.

Raindweller

–1–
I dream in haiku
as it taps at my window
in tart syllables.

–2–
The rain has become
my welcome mat. Most days,
I no longer long for you.

–3–
I soak clothes and skin
in it, bleach private stains,
bury my body's needs.

–4–
Nowhere is it fully
documented how terrifying
it is to be me.

Discalced

I scour the hours you've renounced, trace
the faint trajectory of your absence, ache
for the loneliness of our intimacy—

the ruptured husk of us. I pull the single
boot you've left behind onto the wrong
foot, limping room to room.

This odd caesura of snow, dampening
sounds and scents, milky baby's breath,
crisp white noise inside icy stillness.

How To Write a Poem at Ocean's Edge

I mouth unknowns because there are so many.
I push west from Clallam Bay towards the Pacific,
having left everything nowhere, where it rains,
where it fills my pockets with stones, not shells.

Stones spout long-winded homilies wrapped
in short conjunctions of seaweed. Once submerged, words
are hung to dry. Briny air offers the succinct phrases
needed, rolling along until it delivers, vertex or breech.

I float aimless and unable to swim.
I can't, but I will, I always do. Grey sky drizzles
as I slog along at low tide, stalking verse,
listening as waves compose their capricious syntax.

Mean Distance from the Sun,
Northern Hemisphere, Midwinter

I lie fallow in my eighth decade:
91 million miles
from an imploding fireball
beheld as light
that raced eight minutes
to reach my eyes
and has mercifully allowed me
the miracle
of another breakfast:

       two shiny eggs
       smothered in salsa
       atop a tortilla, pined for
       in preparation, fleeting
       as an orgasm

I sit at a table
three thousand miles from the Florida coast:
a knife, a fork
grasped firmly in two hands
and cut myself
pieces small enough
for a child to swallow.

Nothing is simple.
Not our distance from the sun
nor my distance from my son.

So Much Never Said

If you listen without language, you may hear
my grandfather playing Brahms on the cello,
grunting every now and then with the effort
of an old man soon to die. He played for me

that spring I lay sick with pneumonia.
I was nine and lonely for my mothership,
her planets and galaxies preparing me
for a life of stargazing and solitude.

Although at times I say too much, there is much
I will never say. If you are sad, go to the ocean.
There, is music. Lay your tongue aside, listen.
May you hear the stillness between breakers.

Again I climb

the crest of the last rise
before the road twists its way
downhill to the bay.

She lifts into view, her frosted top floating,
as these Pacific Northwest peaks do,
a mirage above a shimmering cake stand,
and without blush I confess to her—
my dear, dear Mount Baker.

As well I wave blessings to the moon
when it delights me, emerging full
from behind a cloud in leaden sky
to guide me home again.

The me that only sings or cries
alone in the car foresees the day I will not
round this curve again, not drive again,
not see mountaintops again, must leave

home for the sheltered hovels of the old,
fated to never see the moon rise again and again,
and then, to not see again.

Selfie at Deception Pass

You can't say
you didn't know
you would drown here.

There was no deception.
The application clearly stated: "Raindwellers Only."

You didn't come here
planning to jump. You're not a planner.

The bridge soars 180 feet above the narrows.
Click. Clutching at the safety mesh,
buffeted by crosswinds, waters churning below,
you pray an enormous cormorant will swoop down
to bear you away.

You only came here to flee
the voices, to unwind amid
the tall reedy grasses that grow along ponds
and stitch these brackish waterways.

The regret that rises in your throat during the descent
was predictable. Instead of flight, perhaps you should
        have rowed.
The hell that flung you here debarked with you.

Like you, they are only obeying instinct,
seeking arctic shrubs—
these geese flying north in winter.

Last Selfie at Clallam Bay

The car drives to the end of the road, then stops.
The road, once asphalt, has languished into sludge.
The trail, now wetlands, teems with devil's grass.

In the forest, cedar trees peak above low clouds.
They dwarf the firs, which look like perfect
Christmas trees you might find in someone's living room.

The radio dies mid-song.
You drove this road to visit Clallam Bay one last time,
see the bony old fishing village now deserted.

The eagles' nests are empty. *Click.* You may as well shift
into reverse. Take Rt. 112 back to Hwy 101, snaking
the sharp curves around the ancient glacial waters
of Lake Crescent.

When the signal guy waves his flag, you'll know risen waters
have washed out the gravel roads. Here is the place
to abandon cars and phones, time to hike into the woods.

I Am Forest Fire

-1-

Out of dense old growth, ancestors drew me from the
womb, wild and tattered, amidst hectares of organic
matter choking the new. In such an arboreal family, who
could flourish? Thunderstorms, lightning, uprisings in the
underbrush. They said I played with matches. Some said
God. Embers singed the fury of me, left me barren. Who's
to blame? Some flash, others are stricken. When mother
should have been tending, mother was in her lair, smoking.

-2-

Now comes the uncontrolled burn of adolescence.
Incendiary frays that rise to staggering degrees. Struggle for
space scorches the highest branches for a dubious future of
tinder. Don't let the smoke fool you, it's not a mirror.

-3-

A generation dug their ditches, tunneled into earth.
Among razed timbers, seared leavings turned to soil. A
charred rabbit gladly fed herself to a starving coyote. Pine
seeds, covered in pitch, melted, and burst forth saplings.
Two trees forged a bloodline. When I was a young bud,
utterly alone, I envied the others—their beauty, the heights
they garnered. I imagined the blaze of self-immolation.

-4-

The old shall be hewed for a new crop. I'm old now, and
still haven't saved the planet. Hellfire's at the next bend. I
expect I'll fail to keep the promise I once made to burn my
journals—all that paper—before I go to seed.

Apocalypse Selfie

After decades of careening, we landed here,
searching for a feather of hope,
not a head in the oven.

We spend most of our time trying to steer
our solitary ships in the storm. I knew the day would come
when we'd see each other as enemies.

We love what we love, and we hate what we don't love.
Let's just say, *the world is too much with us.*
Or is it, *we are the world?*

When I was seventeen, so many wounded men
told me to smile, my future vanished.
As if a girl's smile could save anyone.

In this town are old and sick ninety-somethings waiting
in their wheelchairs, baggy sweats worn over their Depends,
two World Wars and a bowl of dust to eat
when all the banks failed.
No one tells their stories anymore.

If I were prone to regret,
I'd admit I've failed
to fully love what I love.

We have failed the future.
Our breasts are the drooping ice shelves of Antarctica.
Our gall is burning and brimmed with stones.
Denial hung on our fragile limbs until they snapped.

I hate to close the book with this sad refrain.
I'd rather toast the future, say, *whew, we barely dodged
that one!* But all of Cascadia is burning. It's a miracle.
You can stare right into the sun and not go blind.

Root Rot

I plant clover. I plant monkey grass. I plant simple syrup. Sparrows eat the clover seed and find it good. Mama sparrow plants a nest on my roof and debris plummets down the stove pipe scaring the bejesus out of the cats. In the UK, it's against the law to destroy any sort of bird nest, but in the US, house sparrows "are not protected at any time." A flicker drills house-holes in my loft. I plant catnip. The deer eat the monkey grass. The cats hunker down at the screen door wrangling a sneak-out. The so-very-tiny, ruby-throated hummingbird side-eyes me as she dips into the treacle.

The Daisies Have Returned

It's happening again. Not as metaphor. More like
natural science: first daffodils, then irises and tulips,
the magnificent orange poppies, and now this slight-of-
hand. Will person-blossoms return in autumn? Sprout
new seed-legs from subterranean bulbs? Or rise like
helium balloons released at a child's birthday party? I've
cried every day this month. Forget barefoot summers,
June weddings, senior proms. I long for the rains to start
again. See how blueness performs itself in sky. It's now,
and daisies are exploding everywhere.

And That Is Why There Are No
Origin Stories Anymore

A pair of eagles, twin giraffes, and the two of us
stood there stupidly waiting side by side,
while fish grew wings and flew south
to winter at the tiny ledge of ice
melting the southernmost tip of earth.

Who finds our ruins may wonder
how many millennia it took to heal
swamp grass & redwood trees,
wild goats & floppy-eared elephants.

I want the Ark to stop pairing same-same.
It's not working. Try something new.
Pair the blue whale with a green sea turtle.
Bring back the wooly mammoth.
I'm having that *last-ghost-orchid-feeling* again.
The great flood has come and gone.
Our extinction will nowhere be recorded.

Enough Beauty in This World

Someone on Twitter asks us to recall
the most beautiful place we'd ever seen. I said *Earth*,
because I've never been to another planet.
I'm exhausted & dirty & abandoned &
I still said *Earth*. Floating at the helm of my lonely seabed,
I survey the damage, the centuries of neglect,
& whisper *Earth*. Married to sheepskin, to the elk herd,
to Sundays with only the radio for company, I vow
to love my only mother. I've been handed moments,
small & large. I've wandered many places &
each one stunning: Miami, Kabul, Dubrovnik, Seattle.
I've traveled by plane, by ferry, on the Jetstream.
I've trekked barefoot in ballet flats. I've walked for days
in the desert with only a blanket for water. All of this,
just to remind myself I live here. & still, I say *Earth*.

two

POSTHUMAN

But ask the animals, and they will teach you, or the
birds in the sky, and they will tell you; or speak to the
earth, and it will teach you, or let the fish in the sea
inform you.

—Job 12:7-12

It was a warm day in April when the coleus died.
On the porch, the spider plant bowed its swards
in supplication, scorched by nearby fires. Parched,
the wandering Jew wandered no more. Drought
defiant, the jade and snake plants endured spring,
then died in summer's swelter. The house of wood
quit its joists in stages of rot, and, lost kin of wolves,
a long-eared mutt died inside after lapping the last
scraps from his bowl with a mien of dejection.
In the yard, flies laid eggs in decaying remains;
in due time, maggots arose to cleanse putrid flesh.
And though land lay fallow, ants kept on heaving
100 times their weight to sandy anthills. The bees
were pleased that no one stole their combs.

When humans perish, honey will flow and bees
will grow fat and rejoice. Irises too, when they open
to dew and no boot tramples their wakening. Pink
stripes broadcast the dawn; frogs fall silent; chords
of birdsong rise. The new garden is *posthuman*.
A term I learned from my grandson. We mourn
the loss of Mother Earth but bewail our own deaths
more. Mud will sprout limbs as unnamed flora
and fauna emerge. Until then, we'll fill the birdfeeder.
We deplore human rubbish as if we're not the root
of the problem. We're nearly submerged in waste,
waylaid by pipedreams of time-without-end,
wearing brand new sneakers, t-shirts, and sweats.
Everything I know of love, I've learned from pets.

Everything I know of love, I learned from Tyg.
Today I woke to her face near mine, looking
up at me like an infant at breast gazing into her
mama's eyes. Once I woke to my lover scaling my
bedroom window as I napped in the afternoon.
Such delight, her face. That's not love, yet we swear
by it. Love was being there when my mother died,
racing to the hospital, my prayer she would survive.

I feel that pain. *That* is love. What I feel for Tyg
is a crush—thrilling and effortless. And because she
is a kitten, I confess to something I never knew
in my sordid past of falling in, falling out, falling
over love's devious pathways. It's not love I seek.
It's simple kindness, enfolding me in its regard.

My last lover's eyes regarded me without
kindness. Was it pity? Had I lied or said
something wrong? Was *this* love: that item
I'd ditched on a shelf so long ago? I didn't
stay to discover in her what I'd failed to find
in myself. When Jezebel died, needle in paw,
I met solitude with gratitude. To never again
race home to feed a cat or heed a lover's need.
The earth too, longs to be left alone, impatient
for our extinction, thinks herself an introvert
after all our fuss to clothe her in urban outfit
and edifice. She sends her deep regrets.

Unable to commit, I bring home another cat, and
another. Still wanting a chaste kiss now and then.

I want that kiss right now as I think chastely
of you. The *you* when I was twelve watching
you don a swimsuit, dark nipples nascent
and shy. My first hint of sex. The fine-looking
man I wrote poems to when I was twenty.
That first woman-kiss—on a blanket beneath
a gardenia bush under a full Miami moon.
My mother never kissed me much, or so it
seemed, and my dad perhaps too much. And
when I kiss Tyg, she wrinkles her nose, so
sweet, and licks my hand, a catty-kiss. There
were many kisses in-between, but none rooted.

How hapless I have been! The last time I kissed
a woman, she had a stroke the very next day.

On our last day, the earth will sustain a stroke.
Call it the big one, sixth extinction, apoplexy.
Call it nothing since nothing will be chronicled
on YouTube, on widescreen, in text—only in
sediment. No sentient or sentimental send off.
And not only those who led the brigade, but our
pets and potted plants, the horses in their barns,
the yard chickens we raise for eggs—all will perish
with us. So what if poems make us cry? What good
are tears that won't clean house for our grandkids?
My son stands on the southeast tip of the US
while I hang onto the northwest lip. How long
before highways turn to footprints, feet to clay?
Time is late to prepare for our common fate.

We know we're unprepared for what's in store.
We won't be going home again. What was home
anyway? Wonder Bread and Log Cabin syrup?
Pabst Blue Ribbon and Twinkies? Or was it where
we learned that the birthday balloons we released
did not go to heaven; they killed turtles. We buried
pets in the backyard and fled across continents.
Too late I saw it was I who colonized, sanctioned
slavery, flattened Hiroshima. Our bodies contain
sewage, double lattes, oncogenes. We angst about
the planet and fill our homes with shit. We plug
the ocean with plastic and expect lunch at noon,
milk and crackers at bedtime. Truth time:
we've committed the unforgivable and buried it.

I've committed the unforgiveable. Once,
I swathed a stray cat in an old robe and buried her
in curbside trash. She prowled into my studio
to die nameless. Would it have been different
if she'd had a name? Isn't a dead body proof
enough? I've moved far from that walk-up
in the East Village, far as possible from those
memories. My home is now the left coast, where
I find churning yawns of rising oceans, refugees
drowned at sea, dry riverbeds gone to boneyards.
When strangers come calling, will I feed them?
Will I clothe the naked, comfort the sick, house
the homeless? It's too late to repent. Squalls
lurk nearby. Tsunamis loom at the horizon.

Who drowns in plundering seas?
Who burns in millions of acres blazing
from Arctic to Amazon? Who is bitten by
malaria-carrying mosquitoes newly arrived
in Texas, or mourns the last trumpeter swans'
disappearance from the tundra? "In the end,
the departure came without warning," Etty
Hillesum wrote. *We've* been warned. Before
her murder at Auschwitz, she said, "I don't
think I would feel happy if I were exempted
from what so many others have to suffer."
Of course, I'm unhappy too. Etty rebukes
me, "A hard day, a very hard day. We must
learn to shoulder our common fate."

The common fate of our progeny is to be
left behind as we rise in smoke or choke
the earth with our bodies. Death is a notion
that only occurs in the minds of left-behinds,
as they wait for their own scaffolding to plunge.
Strange days are upon us. Disinterred graves
will float on newborn seas. If you're not already
living the apocalypse, hang on. Soon there'll
be no stone left to unturn, no place to layer
the bodies. No rest, only endless hunting for
potable water, untainted rations. Tears will dry
like barren wells. Soon it will be too hot to
reverse course. Humans to dystopia: "Not today.
Please wait until our generation has passed."

Dystopia has already arrived in Bangladesh.
Sea swallows soar above shrinking coastlands.
Millions of humans are dislodged. Wherever
they roam are snakes, scorpions, wild boar.
In scarcity, all critters are fodder. Some may
test their fins, amphibious. I overhear so much
bullshit all the time, it roars like buckshot,
like a TED talk, like a cop siren. Bad thoughts
invade my mind all day like crickets, like tinnitus,
like hornets. Eons ago, when the seas parted,
Florida emerged. When my great-great-great
granddaughter is born, it will submerge again.
And here I am, on the express train, bypassing
local stops, abandoning her on the platform.

Death will hijack all the local trains, then
round up the laggards on the platforms.
Florida will revert to swamp and gators.
Starfish will perish in subtidal sands while
we stand in the lemming line, marching
in place, sailing one by one over the cliff.
I pray earth will be pleased at our exodus,
its eons of rest to come. In the end, it all
ends—nation-states, Starbucks, galaxies,
the whole shebang. What you grasp for
at end-times hangs on your faith like a fish
on a hook. I envy those whose idea of
the afterlife is taking tea with loved ones
while lolling upon cumulous pillows.

The clouds know there is no heaven,
but are too wise to preach. I wake at dawn
to a private view of fog lifting off the rump
of Port Townsend, revealing the ice cap
of Mount Baker across the choppy bay.
I'll miss the scenery. I tune out the news,
listen instead to the climate moaning in the
wind. Feel the sun's blistering heat. Hum
the dying ballad of bees. There's a code for
what I know but cannot say. How I long
to escape. These selfish thoughts of suicide.
I know death. She'll come in her chariot
soon enough. I'll never cross the threshold
of faith, never know the end of the story.

It's our fate to die before the end of the story.
So I cherish the end of the day, when Tyg
curls up with me in bed and lets me stroke
the bridge of her throat. She purrs, and I feel
blessed. It could be so simple if we planned
time each day to sing in gladness. To purr
at Matins, perform acts of kindness at Lauds,
chant canticles at Vespers. I've longed for
a prayerful life so badly. I leave lakes of tears
on my sheets, never certain if they flow from
rapture or despair. When my mother died,
I thought I was finally free to swallow my
stash of pills. I may not thrive, but I'll try
to survive. At least until my last cat has died.

Nothing will survive. Earth to nations:
"I'm not your green baby-blue anymore.
I'm toxic blue-green algae blooming in
your septic tank." Millions of flushes
ago, when we forgot to prevent climate
change, pond waters turned acidic. At
pH 5, fish eggs stopped hatching. Frogs
died. "But it's no concern of yours, *Human
Beings*." If you are reading this, the worst
hasn't happened yet, even though you are
convinced the worst happened wars ago.
Well, guess what? You were wrong. No
wonder we consider suicide. You only
need the intent, the means, a plan.

Do you have the intent, the means, a plan?
Are you a broken soul? Thinking of suicide?
We want to help. We'll make a safety plan
for you. We're dubious of safety, but fond
of ideation. What's your fancy? Gunowner
with homicidal ideation? Sexual predator
with rape ideation? Racist with genocidal
ideation? It's time to beg forgiveness from
our Mother, she is crushed under our hate.
What's it going to be? Empathy or cruelty?
Teamwork or extinction? Public Service
Announcement: "This is your last debriefing.
We're going off air. From now on, you're on
your own." Name one thing worth living for.

Go ahead. Name one thing worth living for.
Could it be the earth—our breast, giver
of milk and crude oil. Her breasts, like mine,
are empty and dry. In the shower, as I cup
and scrub under them, I recall how they fed
my son, but now hang heavy on my chest.
It's barrenness that makes me cry. Listen
to how Mother groans her death throes. Grief
grows year by year, as friends die of AIDS
or dope, parents are lost to cancer, new plagues
emerge. Until her death, my one thing was
my mother. Today, I'd gladly die for Mother
Earth, confess all my sins and broken promises.
Stop. Think. Mother is tired of all the bullshit.

Mother has lost patience with lackluster
compassion. Birds starve while oceans rise.
My grandsons are now old enough to make
their own babies. And Greta Thunberg
will turn one hundred in 2103. She cares
about a future beyond 2030, tells us that
survival after our departure is *our* nightmare,
but is *her* reality. We stand by as Florida slips
into the sea. No more Viet Nam or Mumbai.
It's too easy to look away, say nothing. Cover
our eyes with stones and lie voiceless under
cold earth. Scatter our ashes in landfill.

Everything needs to change, Greta says.
She's right. Everything needs to change.

Everything *is* changing now. Mama's in the
kitchen warming up human cargo to serve
as leftovers. I dream of trees tapping out new
codes with their roots. We stay the course
as if kismet is right over there, on that other
shore, near the ruins. I turn to you for succor,
but you've disappeared. We're a couple of old
trees separated by loam, losing our lineage.
Beneath bark, youth alter and acclimate.
There will be no further warnings. We must
learn to stop praying for ourselves. High winds
ravage dwellings, wildfires jump canyons,
boatloads of refugees drown as seas take back
the land. Face it. It's not our world anymore.

three

Intuition

As I entered my eighth month
of pregnancy, my grandmother, timeworn
and ripened, exited our line.

Far from home, I received the news
in a whoosh of air, as a warbler trilled
a melody I suddenly understood.

And though there was much to fear,
the awareness settled in me like a deep stream.
She companioned me for the lying-in.

A feral cat crept into the room and stayed
during the long hours of my labor. She
howled as my son crowned, cries louder

than my own, then disappeared. And, just
before he emerged, I reached inside and felt
black curls protecting his soft skull, his fontanel.

At that moment, I received her blessing and saw
his face, still curled in his confinement, and knew,
as a mare knows, it was time to bear down.

I Reside in the House of Her Narrative

after a comment by January O'Neil

Don't ask me about my mother.
Don't tell me to lean towards joy.

Would you tell a dog barking for bone,
a babe bawling for breast to be jubilant?

My mother was not. And so, I am not.
She of the gilded mask and robe,

inscribed with molasses and tobacco. Here,
where sunlight is rationed, I'm the ugly ingrate.

When I pull on the pink slippers and shout:
Look, Ma. I can pirouette, she taps ash.

When I show her my first poem, she
upstages me with her own verse.

Body from body. It's just too fucking intimate.
My infant form faltered, crowned once,

drowned twice. Nearer now to my own line break,
I lean towards the volta. The mother still inserts herself

between couplets. A third foot.
We did our little dance.

I was not chosen. Such a blessing
the dead do not speak.

(This Photo of) My Grandmother

−1−
Whom I forever never met.
Whose lips never brushed my cheek.
Who sings niggunim to me in a language I don't speak.

−2−
Did you know that mother bears sometimes kill their young?
That cichlids brood hatchlings in their mouths?

−3−
I have only this black and white photo. Her eyes are green.
I gaze into those eyes, glance at her slender philtrum.
Do I look like her? I do. I think I do.

She is a wordless blessing, a costume, a gesture.
I swap her headdress for my backwards baseball cap
(black with *Seattle* in pink script). Time and space splinter
into puzzle pieces. Something is always missing.

−4−
Did you know that butterflies drink crocodiles' tears?
Have you seen the mating dance of eagles?

−5−
For what is nameless, I invent—
quaint undergarments,
siblings left behind in Tashkent,
an egg tucked safely inside for my father,
the closing of a book.

Which in time become—
a broken tooth,

an irascible brother,
a love of women,
a silent father,
a father's mother's eyes on a grandson's face.

–6–
Have you seen iguanas fall like coconuts from palm trees?
Or sea turtles go belly-up in the Gulf of Mexico?
Have you ever tried to stare into the sun?

–7–
When you are done, turn the book (the one you hold
in your hands) to page 87 where you'll find
the memo of my death.

Intestate

Start with the cracked teapot. Or the wool blanket,
the never-worn wedding dress with its fluff ruffles.
There is too much, is what. Possessions stain like spilt wine,
objects long rid of stench smell of lilacs.
These are things. Things kept and then forgotten.
In bottomless drawers, bobbins, a thong.
All of this, grounds of a life: Christmas dishtowels
carelessly folded, stacks of photo frames broken,
an empty hourglass. All of this. How the past is a problem
that is never now. How I age and know it.

Sort paperwork, set it aflame, every journal,
all that anguish. It's your great-great-grandchildren
you tarnish now, and no time to make amends.
Get rid of everything you've ever loved
and forgotten. All of it. No one wants it now.
Build your coffin, woman.

At Last I Am Arrived

It took a lifetime to pack, unpack, repack.
        Along the way, I eulogized suicides and cows,

lingered in ghost-crammed cities,
        found solitude in melancholy towns.

Some say it takes an entire life to arrive
        and some never do even at death.

If not dead yet, at least I have a story. But all the yellowed
        leaves tore loose and blew away—

the broadsheets of my leavings. All the wreckage and detritus
        of a life, left behind

to scatter on its own. Every page soiled and trashed.
        I never say goodbye. Look—

I'm dangling a gun from its holster
        ready to argue against another day.

Entering the Gene Pool

A screech owl or flicker woke me.
Perhaps it entered me.

I wait, a watering can
poised above a pot of yellow dahlias.

All the little latencies that have sorted me.
This graph of my mother, that graft from my father.

A lento may break without warning into wild allegro,
while a habit will inhabit its habitat.

Differences are a spit of chromosomes—
a breakup, a split, a mutation.

Arctic ice rolls south, burying
a biome under earth's crust.

The change in me happened suddenly. Overnight.
One day. A millennium. I can't remember.

For the fawn

had no body odor and lay motionless
beside the dead doe, and so
you took her home and fed her goat's milk.

This you did: collared and tethered her, a pet
wandering a yard strewn with cars on blocks
and old oil tanks.

Your darling: adopted, broken, stroked, chosen.
And who am I, who shadowed not her own mother,
nor knows how she is meant to be—
trussed and bound to a fault line.

Remembering Rachel Carson

She had always thought of herself as a poet of the sea.
—Jill Lepore, The New Yorker 3/26/18

I'm on the couch, paging through the *New Yorker*
while the radio is recalling RFK breaking the news in
Indianapolis. City of statues with arms. Reaching. I
cry while Bo kneads my shoulder. I tell him the story
of bringing him in from the rain. Next page, I stumble
smack into the eyes of Rachel Carson. *Poet of the sea.* My
dad used to say, *look me in the eye when you speak to me.*
I can't see eye-to-eye with anyone anymore. Most eyes are
dead and I'm not brave enough. So what's worth crying
over? I can't revive my dad or MLK, all my corpses, the
homeless sleeping in parks under statues, the ruined
earth, Rachel Carson's eyes. I can't stop the rain, so I let it
hide my tears. I've learned to dwell within its providence.
It's all happening too fast. Let the sea have her way.

"My Body's in Trouble" *

I was in the kitchen chopping onions the first time I heard
Jeff's cover of *Hallelujah* burst forth from the radio and land
a blow to my sternum. I lived in the East Village when he
was playing the clubs down there, but I was busy watching
a generation die of AIDS and never caught his act. Can you
say which is worse: Jeff's drowning, your best friend dying
of AIDS, or your girlfriend dumping you two days after the
funeral? His voice entered me like a hollow bullet exploding.
A *broken hallelujah* spew from my lips. My arms raised like
church. I began to howl. My eyes stung like wasps. *You don't
know what love is* rose up in my throat as the knife sliced.

Lyrics: Mary Margaret O'Hara, Leonard Cohen, Chet Baker

Nostalgia Is an Illness You Might Die Of

Last winter I lit a candle, placed it in the window
to guide the night birds to me so I could sleep.
Morning now. I face a slice of pink sky and await
words, dormant bulbs interred in dirt. Your absence
invades my slumber, I will die of it. The rawness
is too much. The final verdict was disclosed
as the blinds were closing, closed. Do you remember
the rough-hewn table where we speared pears
and dared lay slices in each other's mouths
with the knife? Maybe you believe in angels still.

I should ask for help—
a kiss, a pill.

After the Dentist

I slip into a lusterless bistro and order oysters.
I'm always wishing people would just shut up.
It's 2:45 and I was foolishly hoping to be alone.

Passing thoughts are couplets uncaptured, run aground
by conversations I've no choice but to catch.
I want a quiet that tastes like slices of lemon
floating on arctic sea.

When the waitress doesn't bring bread, I don't eat bread.
I'm not interested in intercourse. I lost custody of my son
when he was barely five. I've learned to do without.

I always return to the written word. It lasts longer
and leaves a better trace. I'm not lost out here
in my small craft. I'm writing, not lonely.

Note to Sonia on Her Wedding Day

Like any newborn, he arrived damp
     and umbilicated,

lathered with vernix and swathed
     in lanugo.

On this, your nuptial day,
     I gift him to you.

Though he was never mine,
     I gift him to you.

Today he wears a diadem
     that obscures any remnant

of the fontanel I once bathed
     with such care.

four

Selfie at Seventeen

–1–

Like a blade, it stabbed me to the root.
Rammed my jaw into a concrete wall.
Throbbed me senseless.

Seventeen and broke. Went to the free clinic.
Said, *please take this damn tooth out of my mouth.*
And he said, *first you give me a blow job.*

With that mouth. And I did.

–2–

After the drug deal gone well,
he bought me a bloody steak,
left the waitress
a crisp one-hundred-dollar bill.

How I could have used it!
I vomited all night.
I would never eat meat again.
He didn't even pay for the abortion.

Losing You

–1–
The whole year my son was seven,
when it was time to say goodbye,
we both tried not to cry.

All he said every time
he went back to his dad was:
Goodbye, I'll never see you again.

–2–
You leave a message on Instagram.
I remember looking for you at every moonrise.
I write, *me too.*

It was sweet pretend.
When we ate blackberries and pecans on threadbare cotton
under a live oak. When you lined up your tiny shoes
on the bed, said, *shoe-shoe train.* When we sang our song
about the Milky Way.

My job to soothe, but times I had to pull
the car off the road to re-compose. I was crushed.
Punched a hole through drywall, fist-throbbing sobs.

–3–
Tallahassee. Miami. Tallahassee. Miami.

–4–
We tell each other's stories.
First as lies, then half-lies.
How truth failed us. How I failed you.
How we say, *it was a long time ago.*
How you learned what you learned.

Selfie Under Four-Top

–1–

I tell you how I hate to cry, then a timer buzzes,
and a newbie angel zips by to clip my wings.
It's the multitudes of small setbacks, so shiny-bright at first,
that plug my atria with plaque. After decades
of psychedelics and athletic sex, I took the bit.
Years passed without once going to the gym. Now I'm so full
of carriage, I might drag you down with me.

–2–

Can you see the young waitress lingering in me?
Pouring cup after cup, while glancing warily
at the man with the menacing stare
idling in the back booth. Imagine her dead
along with seven customers, hiding under a four-top,
taking a final selfie. Watch her offer the shelter
of her body to the baby seated in the highchair—
his baby laugh, so delicious—his spoon banging the cup.

Selfie With AK-47

In the dream, I was walking down Shepherd Street
in the old DC neighborhood. Rowhouses of bricks,
narrow front yards lined with flat-topped boxwoods.

Then I saw the man with the gun. Face of rage.
I crouched low on asphalt when a bullet whipped by.
Whistle and crack. Inching towards death, I crawled

close enough to see his crooked teeth. I tried
to speak of peace, as if I could reach inside and shake
his heart back to life. But I couldn't speak. I raised
my phone to snap a pic. His only words were,
aim, click, aim, click, aim, click

Selfie With Baggage

−1−
I dreamt you went missing, left without luggage:
shelves of history, boxes of curses, memories of dead cats
that grazed in and out of our apartments, a jewel box
of grievances. The horse you saw standing in the field.

−2−
I called the long-distance operator
and got a warning cymbal.
The search party threw in their trowels.

−3−
I always return to that image.
The white mare standing in the field guarding the dead doe.
The way *white mare* echoes *nightmare*.
How I came here to be done with my echoing life.
Tell me again how the earth, with all its living
creatures, its biome of flora, isn't rooting for us.

−4−
The story's what's missing. It's only a negative image.
How *not* like Miami. How *not* like Seattle. How *not* like you.

−5−
I'm making a meadow of my lawn, to hell with the neighbors
who stink eye me when we pass on the road
on daily walks, and only me without a dog.

−6−
You left me dangling by a thread.
But I won't forget how that mare stood her ground
with the dead, with a kind *not* like her own.

This Is Me, Floating a White Flag

for Sammy

when your weight
shoves me
to the ground
a flaccid placard
means nothing to you

it's so normal for me
to say sorry, say uncle
say whatever
all your claims
how everything about me is wrong

at six, my nephew
sat at the dinner table
munching a chicken thigh with two hands
licking butter off salty fingers
being a boy rebuked

waving a hunger flag saying,

but it makes me happy
to be like this

Still Life With Dead Sister

The sister I never had
drops by at odd hours, brings me gifts.
She wears a floppy green garden hat and brings
bouquets of mums and poppies. The mums are yellow,
the poppies, orange. She asks, *why live alone?*
She puts the flowers in a vase. I say, *I like being alone.*

She was stillborn before I was born and haunts
my solitude. The sister I never had haunts my solitude
wearing a floppy green garden. She brings tomatoes
and cucumbers, drops them onto the table with the flowers,
lays down her hat alongside them.

The sister I never had slices tomatoes, sprinkles salt,
and feeds me tomato sandwiches.
She makes tomato sandwiches on plain white bread
with mayonnaise. She spreads the mayo thick.
She sprinkles salt on tomatoes. She sprinkles salt
over her left shoulder. She mimics our grandmother:
Poi, poi, poi, she says. She chastens me,
tells me to forget her, get on with my life.
Every time she comes, she tells me I should not live alone.
She leaves her floppy green hat on the table.

five

The Plague

Back then, we swam
in oceans of sex. Desire was
the vanguard of our lives.
O how I remember.

The Hours

I don't sleep at night. I count the hours until morning.
I wait for my bride to carry me off into the sky.
The hours of night are as useless to me as a paper bag.
I count the minutes until sunrise. I doze a bit by early light.
I do nothing all morning. I need to wake. I need an alarm.
I am alarmed that I do nothing. Even a dead dog does
     something.
I want to do no harm. So, I wait. While I wait
I count my breaths. I run out of air. I'm filled with shame.
Shame displaces wind in my lungs. I wheeze and gasp
for breath. The ticking seconds rebuke me.
I am ashamed of things I should or should not have done.
I take blame for your mistakes.
Isn't this the way it always is? Low hanging fruit?
I count seconds of daylight, by light of day.
All day, I cannot stop eating. I am never full.
At night, I don't eat, I don't sleep, I don't dream.
At nightfall, I undo my face. I count my teeth … *one, two,*
three, four. I count eighteen steps to my bedroom.
The bed upstairs is where I don't sleep.
The bedroom door is warped and lets in moonlight.
All night—wind gusts, hard-falling rain, thunderous
lightning. I count the dark hours, flooded with panic.
I am alone. I am almost old. I am old.
My books and my cats try to comfort me.
I lie awake, ready to greet the Sabbath queen,
her fragrant spices commanding me to rest. Wait.
I know death. She will come to me at night.

The Silence of Small Bones

–1–
In silence, we hear
the unheard utterance—
God language. Shaping a mudra, davening,
bending to earth, keening. Keening
a lullaby to the born-deaf child.
A cobalt blue earring in the tiny pinna.

–2–
The infant in the casket, delivered
too soon. Nothing on the scale,
except those few ounces of soul,

a mother
inconsolable, a gathering
in the vestibule, a holy woman
in her chasuble.

–3–
When I worked in the lab
at the abortion clinic, I blessed every bone.
One day, I saw a tiny cochlea—
that little snail of hearing. Praise to the small, byzantine
ossicles wedded in their sanctum: malleus, incus, stapes.

–4–
Look what I found, I said,
performing the sad-ass job of going through your things
while pigeons cooed in the airshaft. Your voiceless journals.
I still hear your bones as they burn to ash.

Cul-de-sac

–1–

The doe slept on my lawn again this morning,
having shooed her spotted twins to glean their own pastures.
I studied my unshorn yard, my habitat, the dewy grass—
having shooed my own featherless from the nest long ago.

Seemed a quiet morning. Fog rolling in across the bay.
Tomato plants showing off yellow buds. Sunny-sides
for breakfast, chickens cackling in their pen.
My toast dry, my coffee black. Someday I will mow
this rowdy yard, coax my neighbors to speak
to me again. Change rustles the page for a moment—
    a blustery warning.
I stopped by to check on him, my usual, bearing eggs.
The one I call uncle on this friendless cul-de-sac.

–2–

By the time they carried his body to the curb
with flashing lights, neighbors had begun to gather
in the street: shoeless, tank tops, bathrobes.
A dog licked my shin. A girl I'd never seen rambled on
about how he owed her something.

I gave my name to the cop.
I told the story start to finish:
I checked for pulse, for breaths. My lips on his.
I counted one, two, three, all the way to thirty.
They turned off the flashers, pulled the sheet.

The Fragrance of Crushed Fruit

for Mary A.

–1–
Another patient died today.

I know the scent, a scent
I know well, but not at all, crumpled into a promise made
five years ago, when it was time to retire,
to go on at least until she died, never planning
beyond this moment.

I can't describe this feeling—
the way clouds claim nothing as they darken into rain.
I waited expectantly, impatient at times, for suffering
to end, but hers or mine? Does it comfort the family
to say now the heavy lifting is over?
How her longing for heaven softened that bed?

–2–
Tears surprise me today. I've held back so much for so long.
I'm scored along the edge, chest ripe for rending.
Yet haven't I've walked this path before, strewn
with the cloying scent of Easter lilies, my own left-behind
longings? My litany of corpses—dare I count them?

O death: you are not a river, but I have careened your banks
my whole career, studying your silences,
submitting to your elegies.
Another Mary plants her son at my feet
so I will know how deep pain can run.

But who can know the sorrows of another?
I choke over words,

feel the soft stir of her in the air, and isn't this fragrance
her must—the crushed fruit of her?

O death: walking past you, so often I look the other way,
ask the buried to forgive the inelegant clatter of my steps,
beg sunflowers in the field to hide their yellow faces.

I have my stash of powder, the knowledge.
Also patience. Finding something to live for
is my talent, this small raft.

Twenty Years of Dead

—Jon (1956-1993)

There's not a lot of love that isn't brutal, but we

had our East Village dives that didn't open for Sunday
liquid-brunch until 1pm and Monday nights at the G&L
community center where all the boys were cruising and
you hung out with me anyway, and

your pâté, your miraculous leg of lamb, your
hundred layers of filo, and

your ten plagues, the infusions that didn't kill
the germ that killed you, and how

after I met your parents, and
after I found the shoebox of postcards of martyred Saints
and slush pile of short stories you wrote in college,

I read your journals.

I should never have read your journals. Your love
was hilarious and full of grand gestures and
caution tossed, and

Christ how we could talk smart and fast like 2 Jews do,
I could meet up with you after an AA meeting, count
on you to say *good god girl, you need a drink*, because

you knew you were going to die and you could say
things so brainsick as *after I die, I want you to burn
my body in the street and eat my flesh.*

Number 16: A Short Poem Need Not Be Small

from 32 Statements About Poetry by Marvin Bell
with a line from a poem by Mary Jo Bang

A short poem need not be small; it need not be small at all.
Even inside a room with walls and doors, there are two skies,
day and night. And when July blueberries yield
but a thimbleful of crop, they are sweet, and it is enough.
If the sun summons sunflowers to bow their heads in shame;
still, they stand tall. Yet, for me, small was too much.
Nothing was what I wanted.

Rhyme and meter too, may skate in on a lark
for the shortest of rides. But words do nothing
to explain why I loved him
so briefly, or why he died, or how I've lived the decades since,
like a poem writing itself without desire.
There were seven years of binging on highballs,
seven of ceaseless sorrow. Nothing about us was small.
A short poem may charm but explains nothing.
After his death, *nothing was what I wanted.*

Elegy in the ICU

To wake each morning and once again choose to go to work.
To grab a cup and a donut.
To gown up, re-use your N-95, add goggles and gloves.
To feel lacking every time a call bell buzzes.
To be a hand reaching out to say *stay*.
To watch the struggle and the surrender.
To notify the family.
To grip the phone while they sob.
To not cry as you remove the tubes.
To cleanse the body as tenderly as if she were your own
      mother.
To cover her with a crisp white sheet.
Her body now groundless as grace.

"ER Doc Dies in Husband's Arms"

for Frank Gabrin, 3/31/20

The City. Streets are empty now, like you always wished when
you lived here, that month or so of summer with no tourists,
if you could bear the urinous aroma of subway stations. Lofty
buildings split sunrays into angel wings, while you longed for
a sudden shower to cool things off. City where my friends
died in droves in the nineties. Back then, it was jam-packed
with yellow cabs & Doc Martins & Keith Haring. Bistro
patrons spilled onto sidewalks at noon, sipping Bloody Marys.
Sounds of yowling sirens, blaring hip-hop, *what-do-we-
want?* demos, funeral dirges. Today, the city has deflated, and
another gay man dies in his lover's arms.

Neither Pause nor Gaze at What Is Passing

For weeks, she said little,
hummed moans in sweet chords, pale florets blooming
on cheeks, chest, breasts.

So much damage. The eye—
only a glimpse. Bloody, blind, suture-shut, tumor-thrust,
bulging from its socket.
Brain of invisible rocks and shards.
What is this death but a scream?

Mercifully, she sleeps all day.
How easy to discard this garment, she says.
A thousand mouths of saviors sing, but none will take
    her place.

When I come, the good eye opens a slit. Her hand reaches,
touches, finds me.
I've brought the lethal cup.
She gives a smile, a signal—not afraid.

She leans into my shoulder, takes tiny sips.
As she swallows, he looks away,
lest she see his tears with her blind eye.

"Body of Well-known Naturalist
Found in River"

A woman wanders to escape. Her noetic life has dwindled
    down to grandchildren she never sees and a failure
to remember their names. She retains an ossified memory
    of the taxonomy of birds, but has lost her car keys
for the last time. She miss-mates the buttons on her flannel
    jacket. There is no one to straighten it or care,
no one to straighten her affairs—

not the trysts of mid-life, but the sort that bury you
    under piles of mail in your seventies. Physically,
she is strong with steady heart and unburnt lungs;
    she can hike for hours wielding a hand-carved
walking stick, backpack not a burden, canvas for shade
    or to lie upon, enough water for a day. She roams
the path along the river where she knows the flora
    and the pitch of bird calls.

The once-weekly chat with her daughter came this morning
    at ten. She no longer looks forward to these calls, but does
her best to fake it. Pleasantries were tendered and repaid.
    No hint was given of any plan or prayer. In the river,
tiny eyelets open within eddies as she slides from bank
    to current with a splash. She is a perfect pear-shaped
sea-bound droplet.

You Are

after W.H. Auden

You are my kitchen.
I can't make my eggplant dish without you.
You dice the onions so I won't cry.
You strike the match to light the oven.
You are my breakfast.
We drink coffee from jelly jars.
I can't sweep the floors without you here.
You are my critic, my lost amethyst ring, my favorite
berry, the knife that scrapes the pith of me, the toothy grin
of the missing boy on the milk carton, my root beer float.
You are the postcard of Calliope you airmailed
from Mikonos, that other time you left, vowing
to never return. And then, the present of you.
Gifts of brisket, banter, sidesplitting quarrels.
I make rugelach every year on your birthday.
You are my morning shower, my evening biscuit.

Raindweller Learns the Names of Trees

I've learned to tell the fir from the yew, the silver
from the red cedar. At sunrise, there is a thin glint of light
northeastward where I await Mount Baker's frozen specter

careening over Discovery Bay. The lamps of Port
Townsend blink; strands of fog hang over fields.
Peckish deer nibble dandelions. I spare my lawn

for their graze. The squirrels, miniature and rust-bellied,
easily reach the hanging bird seed. I don't try to learn
bird calls, they come to feed and that's enough.

There are rumors of big cats. I've seen two elk—
one stared through me as if she knew my secrets, the other,
roadkill. You once told me my poems are too grim

and I should try my hand at something more pastoral.
I've seen powdered snow on cedars, and I've grown
passably fond of rain. Every day, the clouds amaze.

Elegy on the Mourning of My Death

Elders have stopped reading the news. We dream
        of serious play down on our knees—
cat's eyes, jacks, the kiss that's for keeps.

We know spring will come again and again, but not for us.
        We fill the silence with baskets of laundry
and potsful of soup. We can't reassemble the bones

of our dead or carry chrysanthemums to the cremated.
        We read the old cryptic texts on how
to greet aging. Should we speak or hold our counsel?

We prepare for endings, try to be thankful,
        nap in the afternoon.
We have witnessed far too many loops of history.

The whole lot must be coursework
        for something else—
the way the body is water yet manages not to seem so.

The way an egg could feed a child
        or beget a chicken.
It barely matters now. Still, on that morning,

I pray to wake in my own bed, softly
        wrapped in the praxis
of long having known this day would come.

Then, let my fresh carbon mingle with the coal of my ancestors.

Selfie With Ineffable Joy

I stop a moment to gaze
at the evening sky—its shameless blush.
Feeling small and tremulous,
I stop a moment

to breathe

when really there's no stopping us, screen to screen,
selfie to selfie, daybreak to nightfall, we go and come,
come and go, like bots who win at chess
by following rules but know nothing of kindness.

We never own these fleeting moments of armistice—
those German and British soldiers who laid down arms
and sang carols on Christmas eve
still picked up guns the next morning.
Cows will be milked as usual, all is as usual as we drive
to work in a dissociative state, where music
is a mood steered by chance.

I want to take a chance. Be ineffable.
Steep in secret moments of joy. Some nights,
the sky vault yawns like a sleepy child,
the moon's zipper comes undone,
her bra strap loosens,
and a divine fragrance permeates the dusk.

There is the tiny tingle of an ear pulse
that says death will tuck us all into bed so tenderly.
Hush. You must quiet everything to hear.

Notes

"For the fawn": after reading a news story in which a woman took home an orphaned fawn and raised it as a pet.

"Body of Well-Known Naturalist Found in River" was a found headline in the Bangor Daily News, 8/7/11.

"Selfie at Deception Pass": The bridge at Deception Pass is a quarter mile span of bridges built in 1935 that connect Whidbey Island to Fidalgo Island in Washington state. More than 400 suicides have occurred from this bridge, which stands 180 feet above the treacherous waters below.

"*POSTHUMAN*": The quotes from Etty Hillesum are from *An Interrupted Life: The Diaries, 1941-1943 & Letters from Westerbork* (Henry Holt and Co, 1996). Etty Hillesum died in Auschwitz on November 30, 1943. Greta Thunberg (b. January 3, 2003) is a Swedish environmental activist who has been relentless in challenging governments to take immediate action to address the climate crisis.

Acknowledgments

The author wishes to thank the following online and print journals and publishers who have published original versions of these poems, sometimes with different titles.

Agape Editions: "So Much Never Said"

Academy of American Poets: "Ice Would Suffice"

Anecdote Magazine: "Elegy in the ICU"

Autumn Sky Poetry Daily: "I write in the house of her narrative," "The Hours," "Again I Climb," "Intuition," "Body of Well-Known Naturalist Found in River," "Cul-de-Sac"

blinded by clouds (Hyacinth Girl Press): "Note to Sonia on Her Wedding Day," "Raindweller"

Cultural Daily: "Root Rot," "The Plague"

Empty Mirror: "(This Photo of) My Grandmother"

Escape Into Life: "Discalced," "How to Write a Poem at Ocean's Edge"

Floating Bridge Press: *POSTHUMAN* (Finalist for the 2020 Floating Bridge Chapbook Contest)

Gold Walkman Magazine: "Apocalypse Selfie"

HIV Here and Now: "ER Doc Dies in Husband's Arms"

In My Exam Room (The Lives You Touch Publications): "Raindweller Learns the Names of Trees"

Ithaca Lit Review: "Nostalgia is an Illness You Might Die Of"

JAMA: "Neither Pause nor Gaze at What Is Passing"

Kitchen Table Quarterly: "Intestate"

Lavender Review: "At Last I am Arrived"

Mean Distance From the Sun (Aldrich Press): "After the Dentist," "Mean Distance from the Sun, Mid-Winter, Northern Hemisphere"

Menacing Hedge: "For the Fawn"

Moria: "Remembering Rachel Carson," "The Daisies Have Returned," "Selfie at Deception Pass"

Minyan Magazine: "Enough Beauty in This World," "And That is Why There are No Origin Stories Anymore"

Permafrost: "Extremophile"

Psaltery and Lyre: "Elegy on the Mourning of My Death"

River Mouth Review: "Selfie with Ineffable Joy"

Sein Und Werden: "Selfie Under Four-Top"

slight faith (MoonPath Press): "*My Body's in Trouble*," "Selfie at Seventeen"

Spry: "Twenty Years of Dead"

Sweet Tree Review: "Entering the Gene Pool," "The Fragrance of Crushed Fruit"

Telephone: "Old Trees, Old Lovers : A Postscript"

The Rumpus: "How Two Trees Become a Forest"

Whale Road Review: "Selfie with AK-47"

Thanks

To Lana Ayers and MoonPath Press for bringing my
poems to the page again and to all the editors who have
published my work in your journals and presses. To my
Upper Room poetry sisters for reminding me why I write
poems: Jayne, Kelli, Lauren, and Ronda, and the many
other poets who have held my hand, read my poems,
or offered reasons to keep on keeping on. To Molly and
Lauren who read my poems and gave perfect advice. To
a few good friends who have stayed the course, especially
Mary Beth; and to my family for always being there for
me: Ray, Misha, Sonia, Annie, & Sammy. I am humbled
and grateful for all of the poets, past and present, whose
words have brought me through fire and past despair.
If you've entered and enriched my life, engaged in
meaningful conversation with me, counseled me against
suicide, fed me delicious meals, or treated me with
kindness when there was little to spare, I hope you know
it, and I thank you. And, a super big thanks to all readers
who venture here.

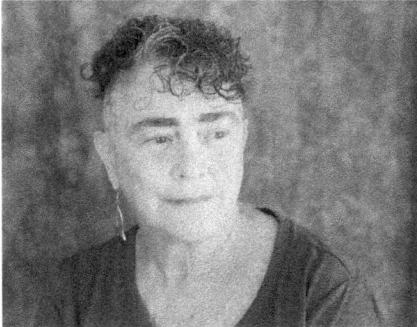

About the Author

Risa Denenberg was born in Washington DC in 1950, and has lived in Miami & Tallahassee Florida, New York City, Kunkletown & Philadelphia Pennsylvania, and has made her home in the Pacific Northwest since 2008. She is a family nurse practitioner who has worked for the past five decades in clinical nursing and education in the areas of abortion care, HIV/AIDS, hospice and palliative care, chronic pain management, and family health. She currently volunteers with the Sequim Free Clinic and with End-of-Life Washington, the advocacy group that supports Washington state's Death with Dignity Law.

Denenberg is a co-founder of Headmistress Press, publisher of lesbian/bi/trans poetry; curates The Poetry Café, an online meeting place where poetry chapbooks are celebrated and reviewed; and is the Reviews Editor at *River Mouth Review*. She has published eight collections of poetry, including the full-length collections *Mean Distance from the Sun* (Kelsay Press, 2014) and *slight faith* (MoonPath Press, 2018), and the chapbook, *POSTHUMAN*, finalist for the Floating Bridge Press Chapbook Contest (2020).

She lives with her cats, Bo and Tyg, in a place of stunning beauty on the Olympic peninsula in Washington state. From her writing desk, she looks out at Discovery Bay and, on a clear day, can see Mount Baker in the distance. She enjoys yoga, cooking, drawing, and reading. She is currently working on a memoir-in-progress: *No Way to Say Goodbye: My Life as a Noncustodial Mom.*

About her writing, she says: *"There is no doubt that my years as a nurse, witnessing illness, suffering, and death, have been the bedrock of my love of poetry. While my own poems are often suffused with sadness and alienation, I am grateful that writing carves out a place for these emotions."*

www.ingramcontent.com/pod-product-compliance
Lightning Source LLC
Chambersburg PA
CBHW032100020426
42335CB00011B/431